Natural Cures for Hair Loss

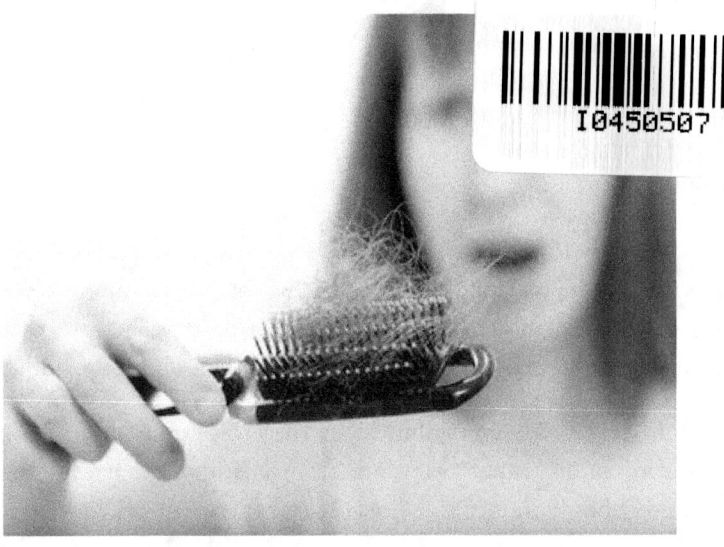

Health Learning Series

M. Usman

Mendon Cottage Books

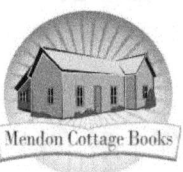

JD-Biz Publishing

Our books are available at

1. Amazon.com
2. Barnes and Noble
3. Itunes
4. Kobo
5. Smashwords
6. Google Play Books

Table of Contents

Introduction

Are you noticing your scalp skin peeping through a handful of hair on your head? Are you tired of finding a clump of hair every morning on your pillow? Does your bathroom crawl with strings of your hair after every bath? Well, you can stop cursing your hair brush for taking away your hair from your scalp, because we are about to change that all.

In this book we present to you a lot of sleek ways to control hair loss and to manage your hair again. Losing hair is not a disease, so don't panic. In the following context, we have traced a solution for you with exceptional vividness.

We assure you that after reading this book, you will be able to appreciate a good volume of hair along your hairline. So, get ready to enjoy thick shiny hair on your scalp waving in the air.

Section 1: All You Need to know

Chapter # 1: Hair Loss: An Overview

In routine, everyone loses hair. Most people shed 100-150 hairs every day. Hair loss is the thinning of hair on scalp. Although hair loss is pretty common, it can be baffling when it comes to your looks.

- **Normal hair fall:**

Losing up to 100 strands of hair is perfectly normal. Therefore, you should not be appalled if this is the case with you. This is because the dropped hair is supplanted by the new hair. It is essential for normal healthy looking hair. So keep on living an anxiety free life with a balanced diet.

- **Need to be worried:**

It is when shedding hair exceeds the number of naturally the growing ones, that you should be worried. About 30-40% of hair density has to be slimmed down to be obtrusive. The medical term for such condition is alopecia. It happens to occur irrespective of age and sex.

Hair loss may include general thinning of hair on the scalp. Some people may experience sudden loosening of hair or bald patches. Some types of hair loss are temporary while others are permanent.

Chapter # 2: Story of Your Hair

Hair is made up of keratin, a protein, and has three parts including a shaft, a root and a follicle. The **shaft** is the visible part of hair whereas the **root** lies below the skin and the **follicle** is from where root originates. Just below the follicle, the hair **bulb** is located. Melanin or hair color pigment is produced in the bulb.

Hair growth cycle can be divided into three phases. Each hair must pass through these phases to shine on your scalp.

- Anagen

- Catagen

- Telogen

- **Anagen – Growth Phase:**

Almost 80-85% of the hair is in this phase is resting lushly on the scalp. Each hair has an age of 5 to 7 years and grows approximately 10% per year.

- **Catagen – Transitional Phase:**

After completing its growing period, hair enters into the catagen phase lasting one to two weeks. In this period, the follicle shrinks separating the skin outgrowth and causing the lower part of hair to get destroyed.

- **Telogen – Resting Phase:**

It is a time for hair to take to a rest. During this period hair doesn't grow, but remains stalked to the follicle. About 15-20% of the hair is in the resting phase. This phase can be assumed as pause before shedding down lasting for 3 months.

At the end of this phase, anagen phase can restart and new hair grows pushing old ones out of the scalp.

The human scalp has 100,000 hairs on average. There is marked variations in the number of hair that a person can lose each day, depending upon density of hair and the length of the hair life cycle. With age, the rate of new hair growth slacks, and any disturbance in the normal life cycle can cause hair to fall.

Chapter # 3: Types of Hair Fall

There are a variety of conditions in which thinning of the hair occurs. Some types of hair fall are due to physical damage to hair, whereas, others are due to scanty hair follicles. In some conditions, only a small area is involved. The following are a few conditions which may cause your anxiety receptors to turn on.

- **Patchy hair loss (Alopecia areata):**

It is a common condition that involves small circular patches of the scalp. Usually, hair re-grows at these patches in a couple of months without any specific treatment. It is an autoimmune disorder, in which the body envies its own hair follicles. It runs in families and has genetic preponderance. This type of hair loss affects both men and women. But ladies, sigh! You are more prone to this evil and it can hit you at any age.

- **Total hair loss (Alopecia totalis):**

It is a condition of complete hair loss of scalp and it usually develops from alopecia areata. The victims are usually children and ladies above the age of 40.

- **Hair loss due to tension (Traction alopecia):**

It is a localized type of hair loss that is caused by too much tension on the hair shaft. Tight ponytails or braids that pull hard on hairs make them fall out of the scalp. Again, this type is common in women. To prevent this, it is better to go for some relaxing hair styles otherwise it will lead to permanent hair loss.

- **Hair loss due to stress (Telogen effluvium):**

In this condition, hair shedding occurs due to premature entry of hair into the resting phase of the growth cycle. This fall out is caused by emotional or physiological stress disturbing the normal growth cycle of hair. Telogen effluvium is generalized hair loss with noticeable thinning of the hair. This is temporary hair loss, especially near the front of the scalp. So women, don't be worried, as your hair will come back. The stressful events may include childbirth, anemia, crash diets and long running illnesses. Sufferers do not need any specific treatment as hair will grow back with the return of the body to a normal state.

- **Hair loss due to mental illness (Trichotillomania):**

It is a disorder in which a person compulsively pulls his or her own hair out or by twisting them, even without realization of this doing. This is the case with anxious or depressive persons. Patchy areas show break off hairs. Psychotherapy is provided for this type of situation.

- **Fungal hair loss (Tinea capitis):**

It is a fungal infection of the scalp that is transmitted by sharing caps and brushes. It mostly affects the children of school going age.

- **Hormonal hair loss (Androgenic alopecia):**

This is also referred to as female-pattern baldness. This condition is often ascribed to family history or genetic predisposition. A combination of genetics and hormones is required for this type of alopecia to develop. Women have the increased risk of this baldness when their hormonal surge becomes turbulent after menopause. This hair loss in women is not specifically along the frontal line but it is a generalized reduction of hair on the crown.

Chapter # 4: What Pulls Your Hair Out Of Scalp?

Whenever you catch a fallen strand of hair, you must be cursing all the factors making it come down. A scalp full of hair is always a crowning glory for any woman, but when it comes to falling hair, this aura turns to bane of life. Often a combination of factors leads to hair loss in females. As a matter of fact of fact females are more prone to be stressed out easily. Here we sum up few of the causes of hair fall to make you more aware of your problem.

- **Dearth of iron:**

Not getting enough iron in the diet can be problematic for you. Low iron in the body means declined hemoglobin production. This dramatically leads to less oxygenation of organs including hair follicles. The lesser the oxygen, the weaker the follicles and its easier for hair to fall down. Therefore, without any doubt, we can say iron deficiency is one of the most common causes of hair breakdown.

- **Life without protein:**

Less protein can make hair fall as proteins are responsible for the growth, look, and strength of hair. So, it is always important to get enough protein. When your body is not receiving an adequate amount of protein, it will shut down the protein supply to the hair follicles. So how can you have hair production without its main structural component?

- **Bad eating habits:**

Your daily intake affects your hair too. Your hairs tell the story of your eating habits. Whether you're taking enough food or not, it does matter. Hair loss is common with those who have poor nutritional intake.

- **Going thin:**

Are you on crash diet to get thin fast? If so, be warned. Crash dieting is one the worst things you can do for the strands on your head. Starving your body of its daily needs just for some worthless beauty purposes throws your hair straight in the bin. Dieting deprives your body of essential nutrients and important building blocks. A body lacking in iron, protein and vitamins will make your hair rough and fragile.

- **Feeling ill:**

Massive hair loss can occur after illnesses like a high grade fever. Falling hair tells you that something is going wrong in your body. This type of hair fall usually follows with hair re-growth.

- **Thyroid want:**

The thyroid secretes important hormones for the development of your body. Whenever there is disturbed functioning of the thyroid, it always has a huge impact on your hair. Hair fall can also be due to the malfunctioning of the thyroid.

- **Menopause:**

A chain of changes happen in the body of a woman when she hits her 40's. One event of this chain can be hair loss. Women of older age should not expect to have a head full of black shiny strands like they used to have in their teens. All this is because of slumping estrogen levels in the body.

- **Blessing of newborn:**

Your baby is indeed a blessing for you. While being busy playing with this angel, you notice a clump of hair wrapped around his or her fingers. If this is so, then relax, as it is normal for this to happen. Hair fall within a few months after delivery is common, and again, this is due to jumping estrogen imbalance in the body. After delivery, estrogen levels crash, throwing hair into the resting phase. This unusual shedding will soon end with new hair growth.

- **Stress:**

What is on your head reflects what is in your head. A physical or emotional shock can lead to general thinning of hair. Tension on your nerves has an impact on your hair growth too.

- **Pharmacy rivals:**

Some medicines disturb the hair growth cycle. These medications can be helpful for cancer, heart diseases, depression and blood pressure but are not favorable for hair. Such drugs also include steroids, birth-control pills, blood thinners, and high doses of vitamin A supplements.

- **Cheaper products:**

Cheaper and inappropriate products for hair can cause excessive hair damage. These products not only make hair lusterless and fragile, but also shorten their life duration. Excessive use of dyes, cheaper hair colors, gels, sprays, and bleaching can cause drastic hair breakage.

- **Hair styling tools:**

Before going to a party or a get together, you just put the flattening iron on to get a sleek straight look, or blow dry your hair with the use of heat. But all this styling tools are high heat that are damaging to your hair. Regular use of an iron can burn your hair making them rough and brittle. Blow dryers can evaporate water from the hair shaft making it dry. All these tools might be good for your look at the get together, but their undue use can make you yell at them.

- **Clip hair styles:**

Holding hair tightly with hair bands and clips can cause unusual hair breakage. Tight high pony tails put a strain on the hair root and pull it out of its follicle.

- **Bad hair manners:**

Aggressive shampooing, combing, or brushing can cause hair to expire from your scalp and come down in your hand. Rubbing wet hair with a towel to make it dry can also cause hair breakage.

Section # 2: Solution to Your Problem

The fear of excessive hair loss or going bald is what usually instigates women to look for medical treatment. This hair loss can be ravaging to their self-esteem. Usually women with a thin crown hesitate to go in public. They tend to cover their head and let not their hair flaunt in air.

This section is especially for those poor women. If you are a sufferer, then stop wasting your time and money on buying expensive hair products that are good for nothing. Just sit down and give a look to the upcoming chapters to have your head full of shiny hair. We assure you can restore your mane by following these simple, but useful, techniques.

Chapter # 1: Give Hot Oils a Try

Hot oil treatments are always effective for reducing hair loss. Massaging your scalp regularly with warm oil, just for few minutes, can perk the circulation up. Maintained circulation to the hair follicles, can help to keep them active and in growing age. Here is a list of oils you can use for regular scalp massage.

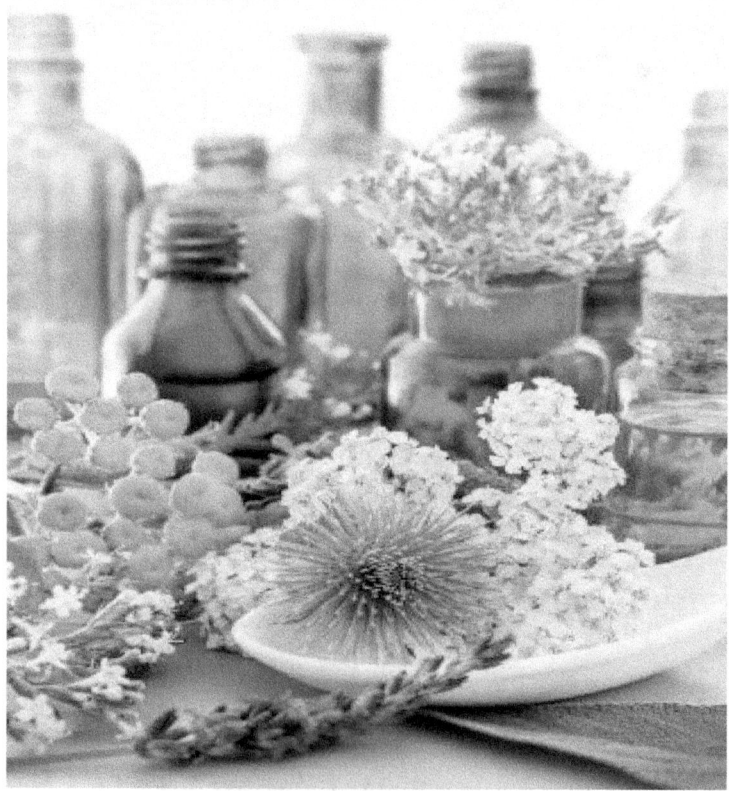

- **Olive oil:**

Olive oil is high in antioxidants including vitamin E and monounsaturated fatty acids that promote hair growth and make them less likely to break. Olive oil penetrates better in the hair shaft and makes it stronger and healthier. It is also an excellent hair conditioner. Massaging your scalp with olive oil for a few minutes nourishes the hair follicles and works for dry, brittle hair.

- **Almond oil:**

Who can deny the benefits of almonds? Almond oil is one of the most nutritious oils when it comes to either intake or external use. Almond oil is rich in vitamin D, E, fats, calcium and magnesium. Moreover, it can be easily absorbed by hair. In addition to its softening action, almond oil also acts as a natural moisturizer. It helps hair to grow faster, thicker and stronger.

- **Coconut oil:**

Coconut oil is probably the best oil for hair. Thicker and healthier hair of its users is proof of its beneficial role for hair loss. Coconut oil prevents hair from losing moisture and keeps them dense and strong. It contains lauric acid, which is an antibacterial agent and helps to keep your scalp infection free.

- **Castor oil:**

If you are searching for some treatments for hair re-growth, then you can use castor oil as a quick scalp treatment. Castor oil is rich in omega 9 fatty acids. It goes deep into the pores of skin and provides nourishment to both hair and the follicles. Castor oil has scalp rejuvenating property thereby increasing circulation to the scalp and promoting hair growth at a faster rate.

- **Rosemary oil:**

Rosemary oil, obtained from rosemary leaves, is often used in shampoos. It has a reputation for stimulating hair growth. It stimulates cell division and dilates the blood vessels. This act, in turn, leads to improved circulation to the scalp enhancing hair growth. Rosemary oil can be mixed with other essential oils to prevent hair loss.

- **Lavender oil:**

Lavender oil has been in use by many cultures for its calming and relaxing properties for ages. It is highly effective against lice, too. Owing to its anti-bacterial action, it keeps the infections away from the scalp.

- **Jojoba oil:**

When it comes to using jojoba oil for hair loss, its users admire its healthy effects. It goes deep into the pores and helps clogged pores to throw excess sebum and other impurities out. In this way it promotes hair growth. It also hydrates the hair strands making them shiny and vibrant. It is an excellent emollient for dry damaged hair and provides protection against high heat of hair styling tools and harmful sun rays.

- **Cedar wood oil:**

If you have cedar wood oil among your hair loss prescription then wave bye-bye to damaged hair. Cedar wood oil has long history of its use for hair loss, dandruff and itching. It acts as anti-seborrhoeic and tonic and is beneficial in curing inflammatory diseases of scalp.

- **Thyme oil:**

Thyme oil is helpful for new hair growth and slowing down the hair fall process. Thyme oil is very good for turning hair into healthier and denser one. It can also be used in the mixtures of oils for hair loss.

- **Chamomile oil:**

Chamomile oil is soothing for the scalp and is known for its nerves calming ability. It is highly effective for dry, brittle hair. It kills lice and makes hair free of this blood sucker. Chamomile oil provides protection to hairs against harsh environment and help with itching and dandruff.

- **Peppermint oil:**

Peppermint oil is high in the ranks for improving blood circulation to the hair roots and thus promoting hair growth. It is also refreshing and rejuvenating for the scalp. Healthy hair follicles owe their existence to peppermint oil.

- **Combinations of oils:**

Mixture of oils are always a way to go for hair loss, hair re-growth and for better looking hair.

Mixture # 1:

For this you need 15 ml of apple cider vinegar, 6 drops of rosemary oil, and 6 drops of jojoba oil, 3 drops of geranium oil, 50 ml of rosewater and 50 ml of distilled water. Mix all these oils and water and shake well. Use it after washing your hair with mild shampoo.

Mixture # 2:

Mix equal quantities of castor oil and almond oil in a clean container. Apply this mixture to the areas of thinning. Use with wet fingers for easy application and spread. Apply it for a night and then rinse it off. This mixture is best for hair re-growth.

Mixture # 3:

Add 2 tablespoons of olive oil and 2 tablespoons of coconut oil to 1 tablespoon of aloe vera gel. Blend this mixture and apply on the scalp for 20 minutes. Rinse it off with any suitable shampoo.

- **Hair masks:**

Hair masks work for conditioning and moisturizing the hair. These masks can be applied any time to get shiny, lustrous dense hair.

Mask # 1:

Mix egg white, 2 tablespoons of curd, and 2 teaspoons of olive oil. Apply this mask to your scalp and hair for 20 minutes. Rinse it off. You will feel extremely smooth and silky hair on your top.

Mask # 2:

Mash a banana. Add 2 teaspoon of olive oil or jojoba oil to this. Apply the mixture to the scalp for 15 minutes. Shampoo your hair and let it flaunt.

Chapter # 2: Go Grab Herbs

Herbs have a wide variety of actions that can be beneficial for the skin, immune system, metabolic system, and hair. Side effects of medicines and chemical products make the worried users shift their attention to all natural treatments, and nothing is more natural than herbs. If you are also searching for some natural treatments for hair loss, then you have clicked the right option. The following chapter gives you an enormous knowledge of herbs that worth your attention.

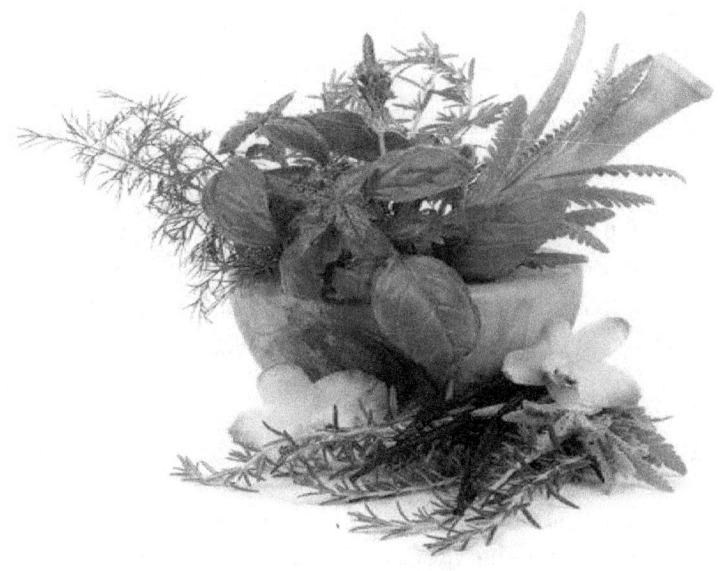

- **Henna:**

Being known as a natural hair color and hair conditioner, henna is helpful in strengthening hair strands.

How to use:

Mix 1 cup of dried powder of henna leaves with half cup of curd. Apply this mixture to hair and allow it to dry. After one hour, wash your hair with mild shampoo. You will feel silky shiny strands of hair waving in the air.

- **Aloe Vera:**

This herb, in gel form, helps to restore hair growth and thickness. The ancient Egyptian medicine people used Aloe Vera to reduce hair loss. Aloe Vera removes dead cells from the scalp, helping open the clogged pores. This will lead to improved nutrition to the follicles and enhanced hair growth. It also balances the pH of scalp at optimum level for hair growth.

How to use:

You can use Aloe Vera gel directly on scalp. Leave it on for 2 hours and then rinse it off with mild shampoo.

You can prepare hair mask by mixing half cup of Aloe Vera with 2 tablespoons of castor oil and 2 tablespoons of fenugreek powder. Apply this mixture to your scalp and leave it overnight. In the morning wash it with a mild shampoo. The volume of hair can be increased massively by regularly using this mask once a week.

- **Amla:**

Amla is a perfect solution for most hair loss sufferings. This herb is packed with antioxidants including vitamin E, C, vitamin B complex and also with calcium, iron and phosphorous. It promotes hair strength and gives more shine to the fine threads on your head.

How to use:

Use amla and shikakai in 1:1 ratio. Mix them well and make a paste. Apply this paste to your scalp and let it dry for a few minutes and then wash with any suitable shampoo.

You can also mix two teaspoons of amla powder with equal quantity of freshly squeezed lemon juice. Apply the mixture to the scalp and leave to dry. Wash it afterwards with lukewarm water.

- **Neem:**

Neem reduces hair loss by stabilizing the hair thinning process and then strengthening them. It also has anti-bacterial action helping itching and dandruff prone scalps.

How to use:

Boil Neem leaves in sufficient water until water dries to half of its quantity. Rinse your hair with this water once a week.

- **Bhringaraj:**

Bhringaraj is a main component of hair tonics for preventing hair loss and is a known medicine for baldness. It also prevents premature graying of hair.

How to use:

Get 50 grams of Bhringaraj leaves and crush or grind them. Boil 200 ml of coconut oil in a pan. Add these crushed leaves along with 2 teaspoons of fenugreek seeds into the boiling oil. Let the mixture boil for 10 to 15 minutes until you notice bubbles of oil forming in the pan. Remove the pan from the flame and leave it for a night, covered. With the sun rise, strain this oil into a glass jar or any container and put it aside for regular use.

- **Ginseng:**

You might have read this word on the packing of homeopathic medicines for hair or skin. It has been used in Chinese medicines for years because of its well-known beneficial effects. Ginseng enhances the proliferation of skin cells encouraging regeneration of hair follicles.

How to use:

You can obtain ginseng oil by boiling ginseng herb in tea tree oil for a sufficient time. Use this preparation regularly and you will notice the difference.

Chapter # 3: Be Rich for Food

"Just like every other part of your body, the cells and processes that support strong, vibrant hair depend on a balanced diet," says New York nutritionist Lisa Drayer, MA, RD, author of *The Beauty Diet*. If you want shiny thicker hair, then you must have a look at the nutrients you are taking in. What you take in is exactly the same as what your hair gets. Keep your diet in check and enjoy a fuller thicker mane. No one can have more of the crowning glory as he or she used to have at the time of birth. Only diet can enhance the beauty and health of hair for your better and glamorous look. Here are some diet tips for you to get rid of the panicking hair strands in the brush.

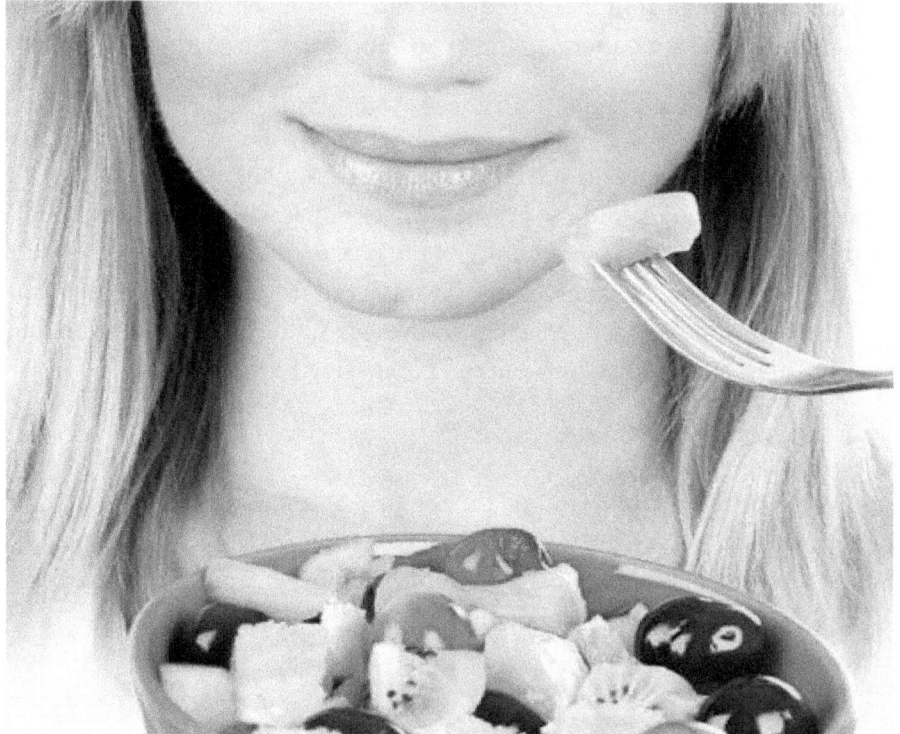

- **Pack your food with protein:**

The building component of hair is protein, so you must ensure adequate intake of protein for the growth of hair. If your protein stores are depleting, then you will end with up having brittle and lusterless hair. Here is a list of protein packs to fulfill your thicker hair dream.

> ### *Eggs:*

Eggs are undoubtedly the greatest source of protein. In addition to this, they are also rich in selenium, iron, sulfur and zinc. Greet your rising sun with healthy eggs in your breakfast. You can have this protein pack as a mask on your head too.

> ### *Meat:*

Let me tell you vegetarians, you are skipping a huge deck of proteins in the form meat. Cook chicken and turkey to have them for your hair.

> ### *Lentils:*

Lentils are the vegetarian source of proteins along with iron. These include starchy beans, kidney beans, and black-eyed beans. Toss these tiny but mighty beans in your salad or soup to get a boost of biotin as well.

> ### *Yogurt:*

Yogurt is a hair friendly protein. Cottage cheese and low fat cheese also come in under this category. You can cherish your taste buds with these nutritious ingredients at any time. But you can cover your hair strands with them too.

- ### Fill the fist with essential fatty acids:

No girl will want to run her fingers through dull and dry hair. To escape this, you have to have essential fatty acids in your diet. What these fatty acids do is to condition and nourish your body and hair as well.

> ### *Walnuts:*

When it comes to food that gives you a beauty punch, it is hard to skip walnuts. Walnuts are a terrific source of omega-3 fatty acids along with selenium and zinc. Having walnuts regularly is the best way to fight hair loss. If you don't have these fatty acid rich fighters in your diet, your hair will snap.

➢ *Salmon:*

Have you ever tried salmon for thick, shiny hair? You should, as it is loaded with high quality proteins, omega-3 fatty acid, iron and vitamin B-12. What can give you more nutrition than this? It keeps the scalp well hydrated, so vegetarians don't hesitate to put this tiny cold water creature on your platter.

- **Eat iron:**

Iron is essential for hair growth and strength. Low iron levels can lead to anemia which in turn leads to hair loss. In anemia, the nutrient supply to follicles is disrupted, causing a disturbed hair growth cycle. This follows with the shedding of hair. Lentils and green leafy vegetables are rich sources of iron.

➢ *Spinach:*

Spinach is rich in iron, beta carotene, vitamin C and folate. All these vitamins and minerals keep good circulation to the scalp and enhance hair growth.

- **Work up with vitamin C, E and A:**

Vitamin C ramps up the collagen production around hair strands, making them strong and less vulnerable to breakage. Vitamin C rich foods are blueberries, strawberries, kiwi fruit and oranges. Vitamin E is required to nourish damaged hair. It helps the body to produce keratin which means it helps in the development of each hair strand. Vitamin E is contained in egg yolks and nuts. Vitamin A is required by the body to produce sebum. Boosting our hair's oily sebaceous glands, it helps to condition our hair. Without sebum, the scalp will go dry and itchy. Vitamin A rich foods are sweet potatoes, pumpkins and carrots.

➢ *Blueberries:*

It is a nutrient super fruit for vitamin C. To get enough of vitamin C, you can't skip this exotic fruit. It supports blood vessels to restore circulation to feed the hair follicles.

> ➤ *Sweet potatoes:*

Sweet potatoes are rich in beta carotene, a precursor of vitamin A. you can never have too much of good things when it comes to vitamin A, as it performs many important functions in our body. It keeps the oil production high in the scalp to keep it conditioned.

Chapter # 4: Set Free Your Stressors

You have to believe this fact that most of the time, the root cause of hair fall is stress and tension on your nerves. When everything is alright including your diet and hair care, then what you need to do is to find your stressor and give it a bash. Your stress is unique to you and you have to search for a suitable way to eliminate it.

- **Take a deep breath:**

It is the best and easiest technique that can be done anywhere at any time. Give yourself just a five minute break, close your eyes, sit straight and focus on how the air fills your insides and goes out. It is the simplest way to make your head lighter.

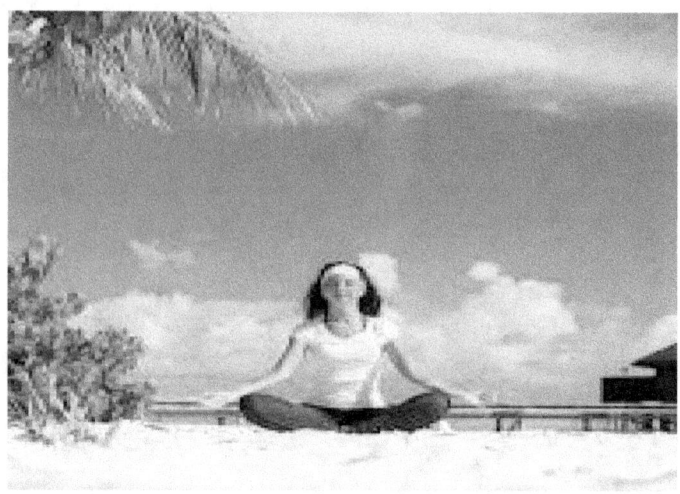

- **Hit the walking track:**

Mild to moderate exercise keeps your body away from tensing chemicals. Exercise keeps you healthy and fresh. What it has to do with hair is enhanced circulation and blood flow encouraging hair growth.

- **Practice meditation:**

You don't need to empty your pockets out at meditation. Meditation focuses your attention and releases entangled strands of thoughts. It is helpful not only for emotional, but also for physical stability including what you have on your head.

Prevention and conclusion

Taking good care of anything actually maintains it and prevents its disruption. This is true for hair too! Girls often don't give attention to their hair until they feel drastic hair loss by noticing entangled hairs in the comb. It is always better to start early care before it's too late. To prevent hair loss, you have to develop good hair care habits. Make a suitable cleaning plan for hair. Do not give space to harsh chemicals for coloring or styling your hair and treat your hair just like a princess. Following are some preventive suggestions for reducing your hair fall.

- Keep your hair away from the high heat of styling tools. Heat weakens hair proteins leading to hair-loss. Thus hair dryers, hot curlers, and hair irons should be used very seldom, if at all.

- Don't ruin your hair just for the sake of hurry. Don't ever comb wet hair. Relax; give them time to get air dried. Also use a wide toothed comb and brushes with soft bristles. This will prevent clumps of hairs entangling in hair brush.

- Avoid tight low quality rubber bands, or elastics on your hair. Tightly done hair styles can cause breakage and ultimately hair loss. To prevent hair loss, it is always better to avoid tight ponytails or braids.

By simply following the above tips along with diet and exercise, you'll feel how simple it is to pamper your hair. Give your hair a little bit of your time and your attention instead of spending a lot of money on it.

Author Bio

Muhammad Usman is a distinguished medical graduate of Allama iqbal medical college (AIMC). He is a professional writer who has been in the field for more than 4 years. During this time he has produced 10,000+ articles, blogs and eBooks on various niches related to diseases, health, fitness, nutrition and well-being. He is a regular contributor to several journals related to medicine and surgery. He is the editor of several journals and newspapers.

Check out some of the other JD-Biz Publishing books

Gardening Series on Amazon

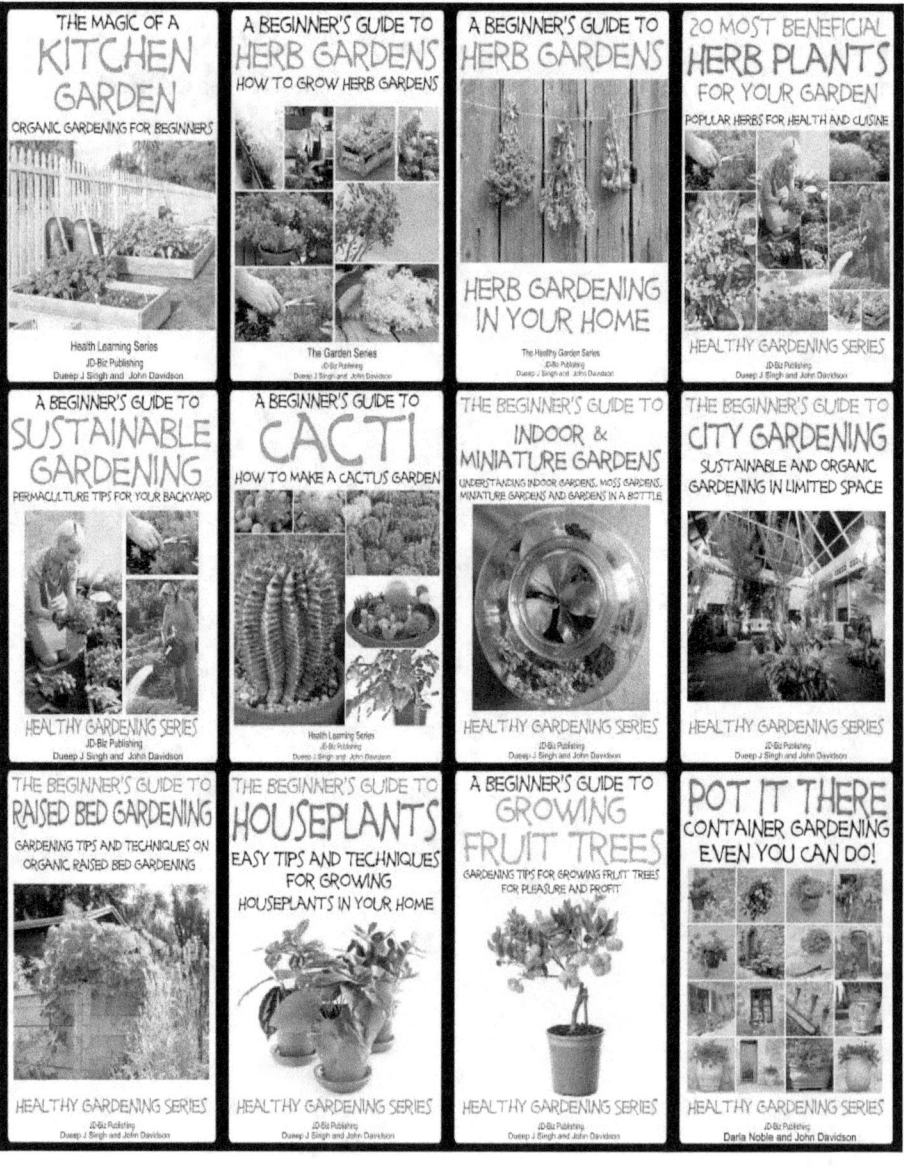

Health Learning Series

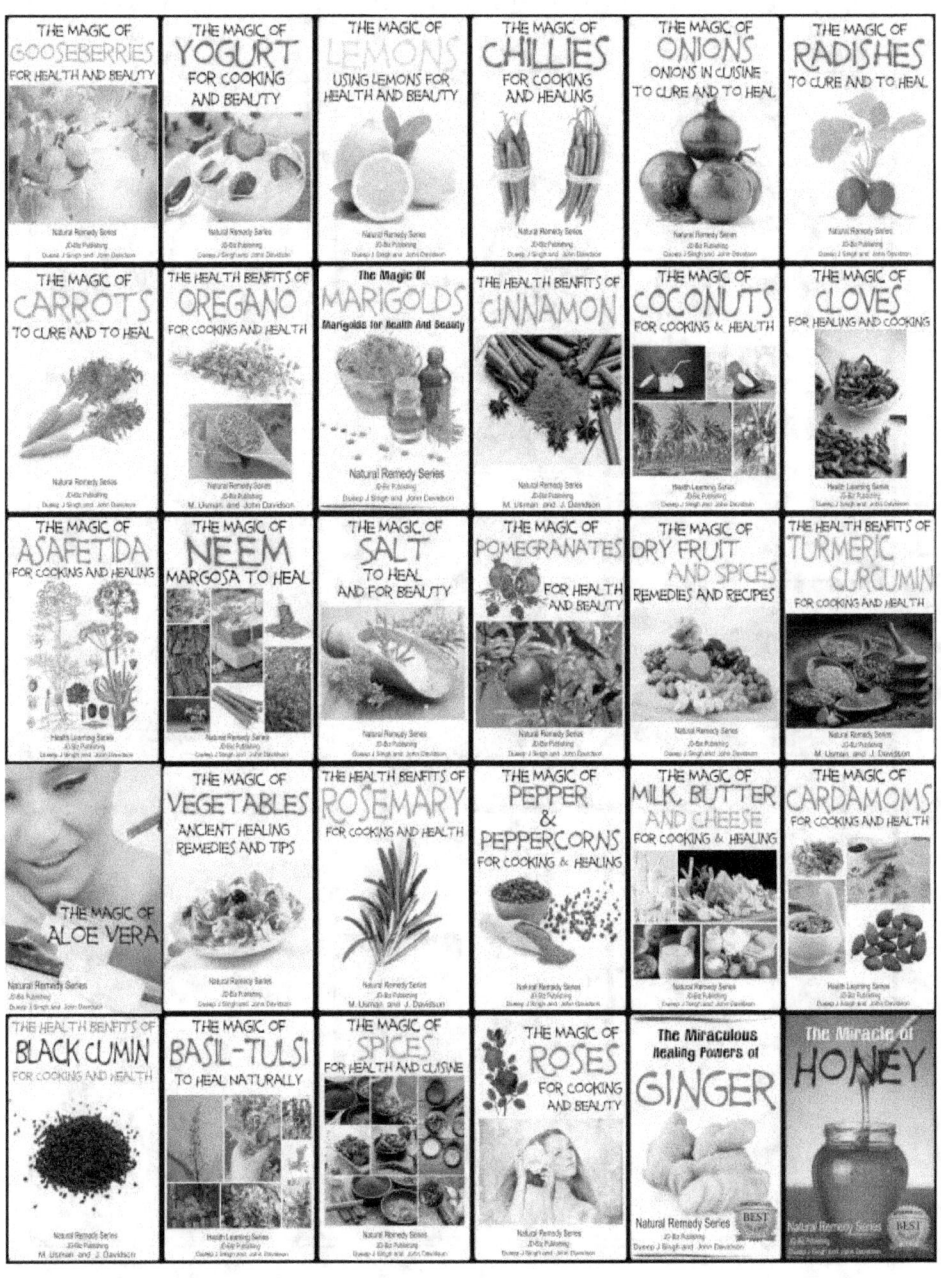

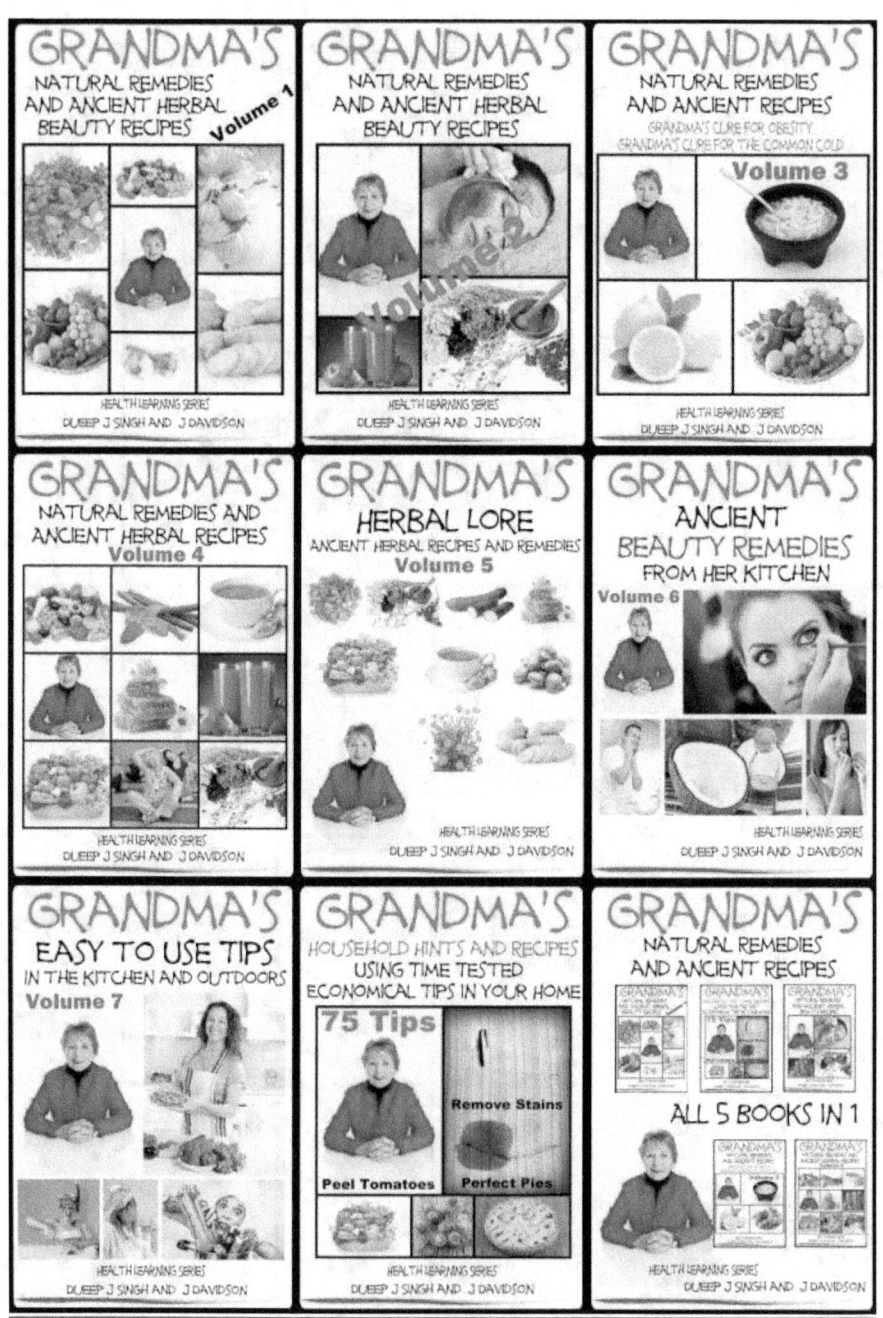

Country Life Books

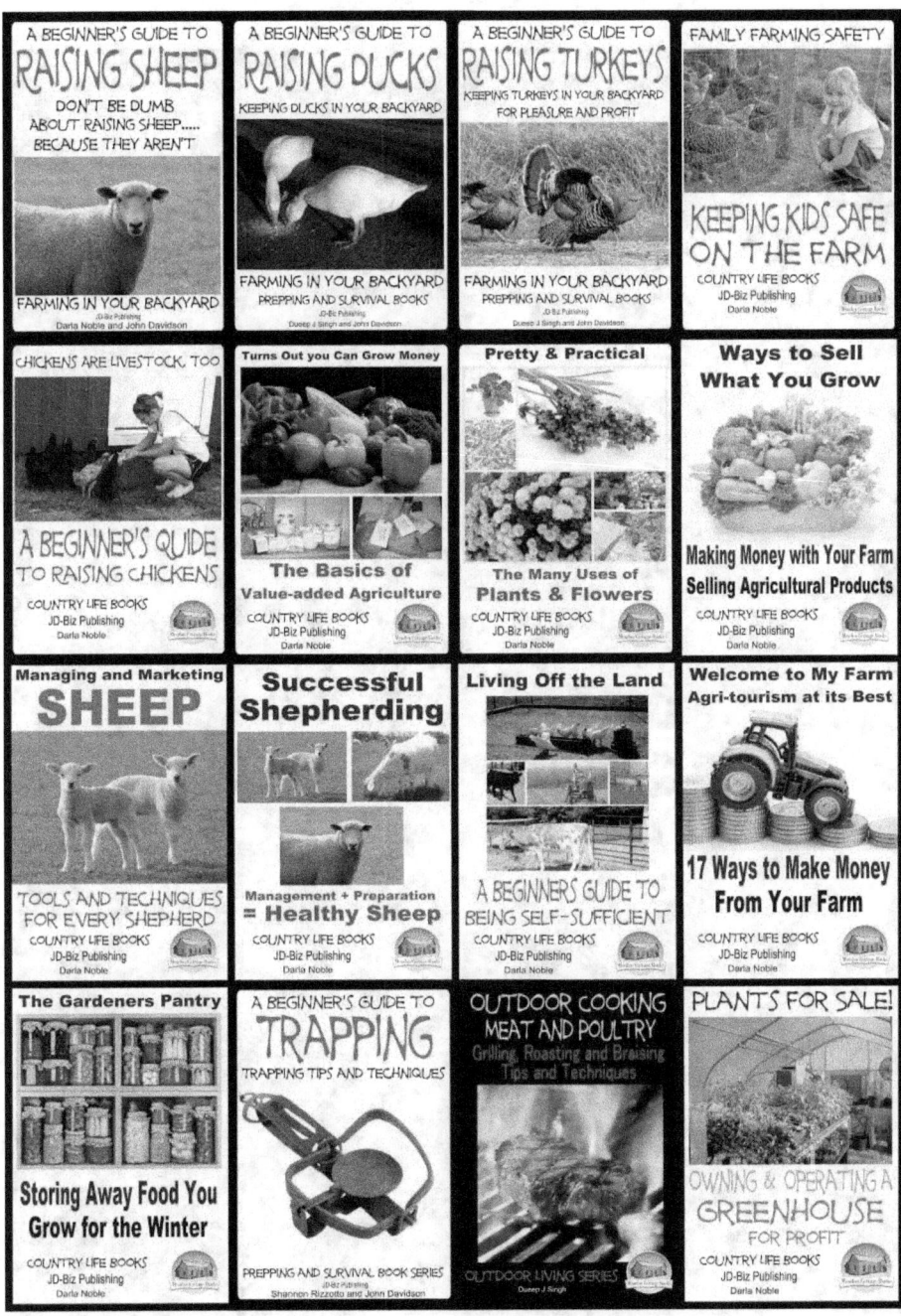

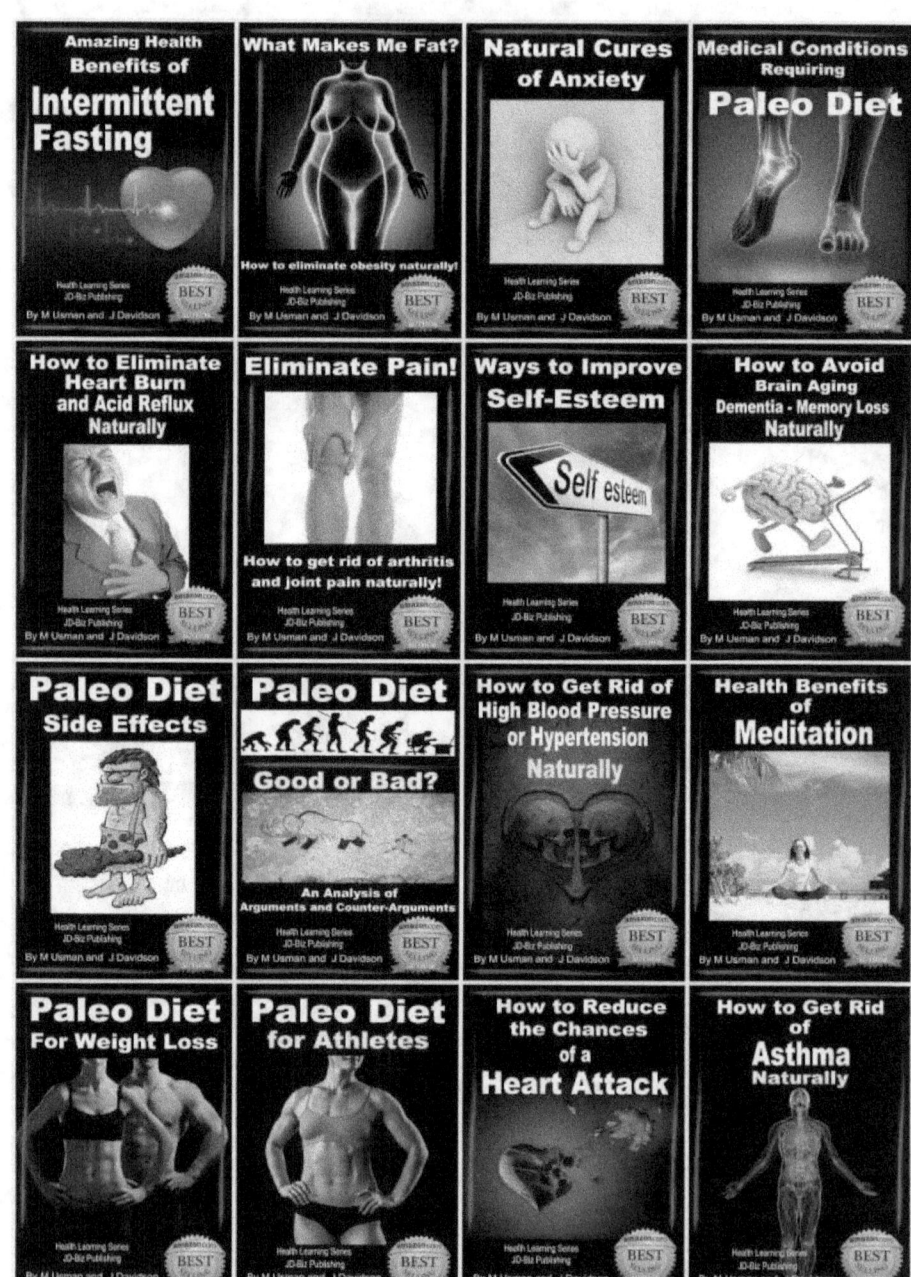

Amazing Animal Book Series

Chinchillas · Beavers · Snakes · Dolphins · Wolves · Walruses

Polar Bears · Turtles · Bees · Frogs · Horses · Monkeys

Dinosaurs · Sharks · Whales · Spiders · Big Cats · Big Mammals of Yellowstone

Animals of Australia · Sasquatch - Yeti Abominable Snowman Bigfoot · Giant Panda Bears · Kittens · Komodo Dragons · Lady Bugs

Animals of North America · Meerkats · Birds of North America · Penguins · Hamsters · Elephants

Learn To Draw Series

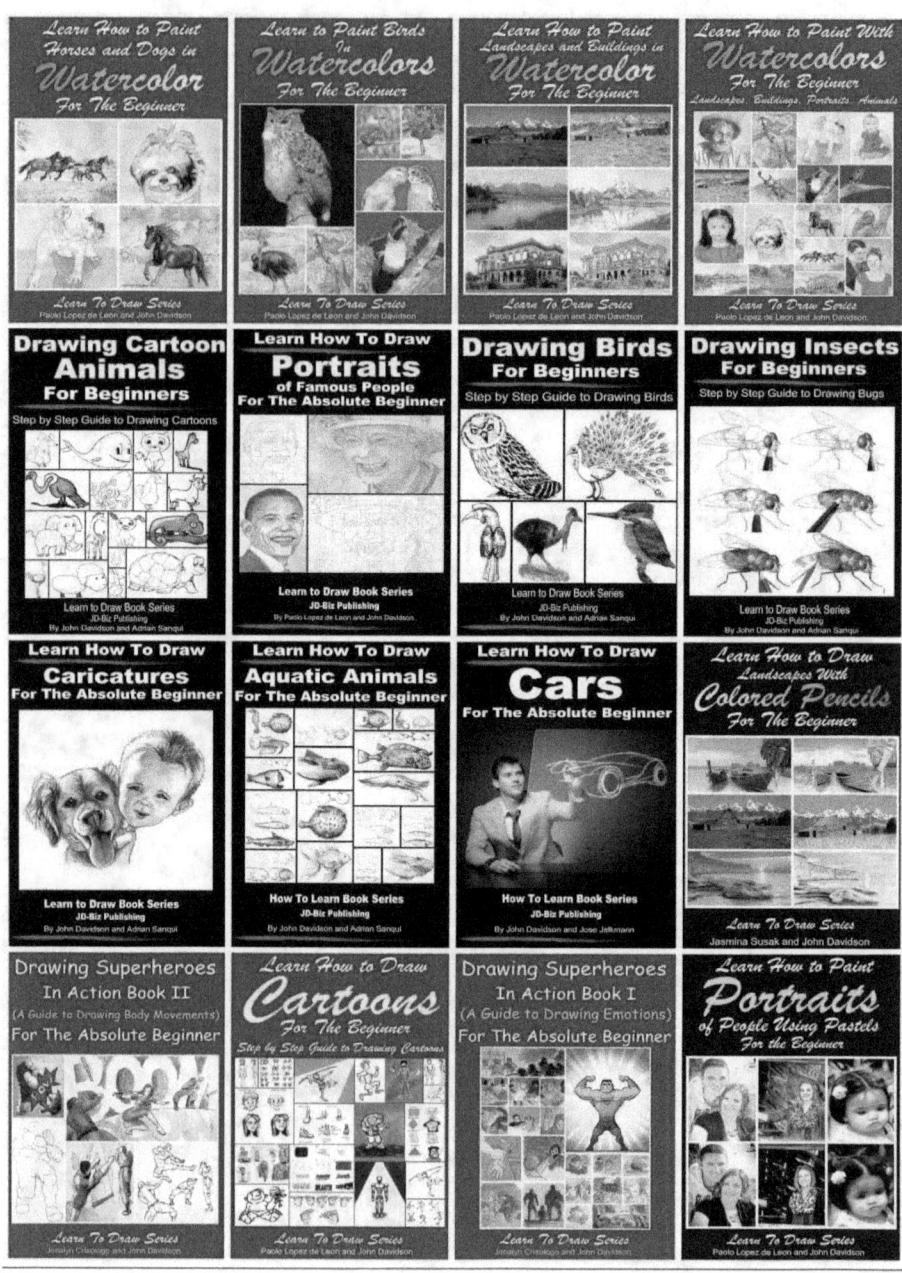

How to Build and Plan Books

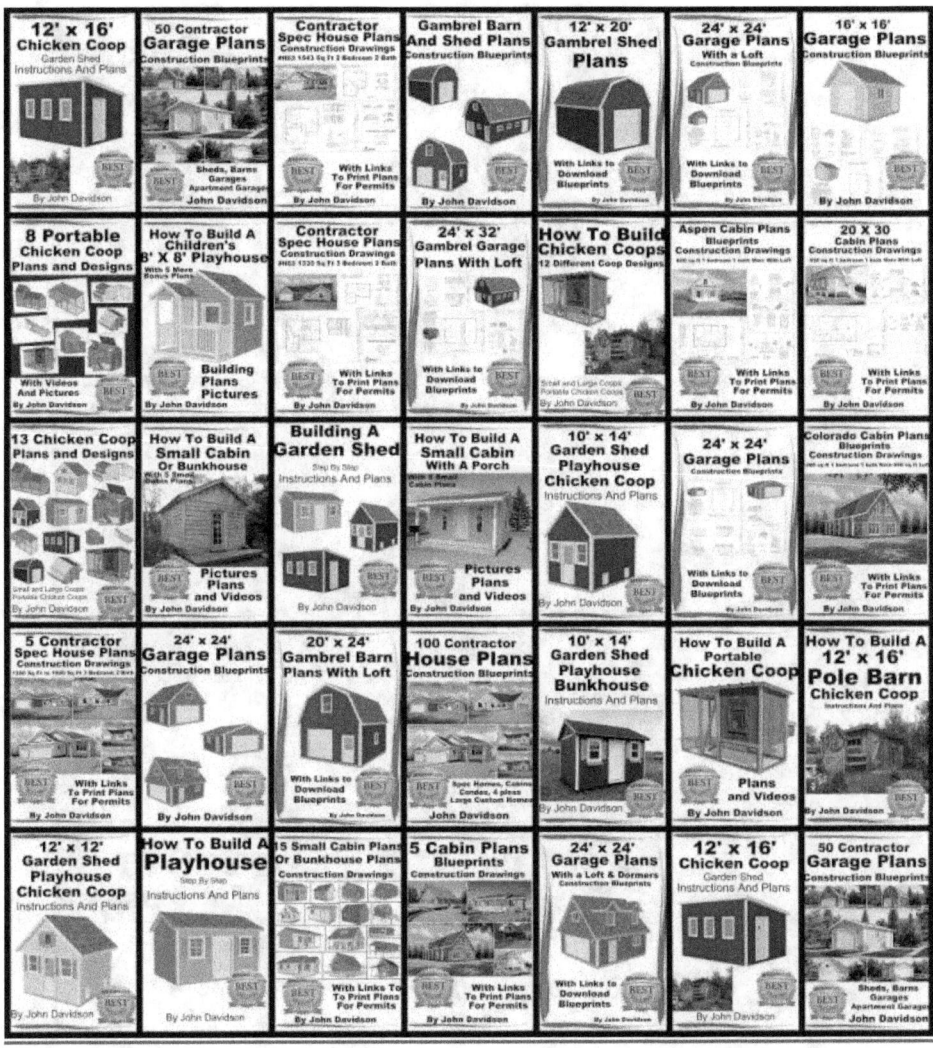

Entrepreneur Book Series

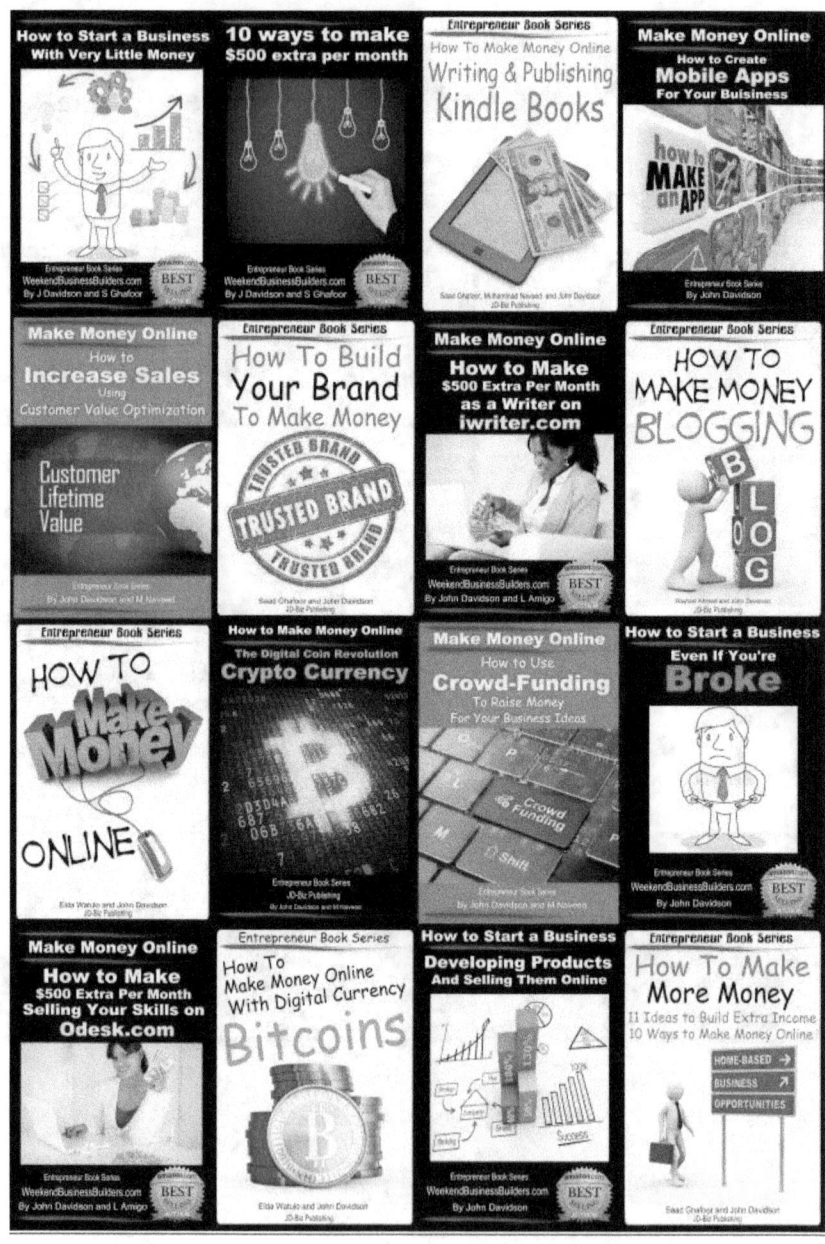

Our books are available at

1. Amazon.com

2. Barnes and Noble

3. Itunes

4. Kobo

5. Smashwords

6. Google Play Books

Publisher

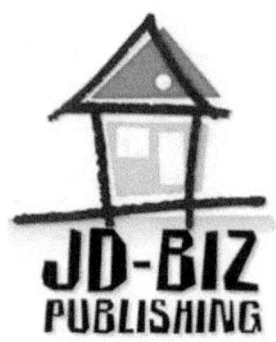

JD-Biz Corp

P O Box 374

Mendon, Utah 84325

http://www.jd-biz.com/

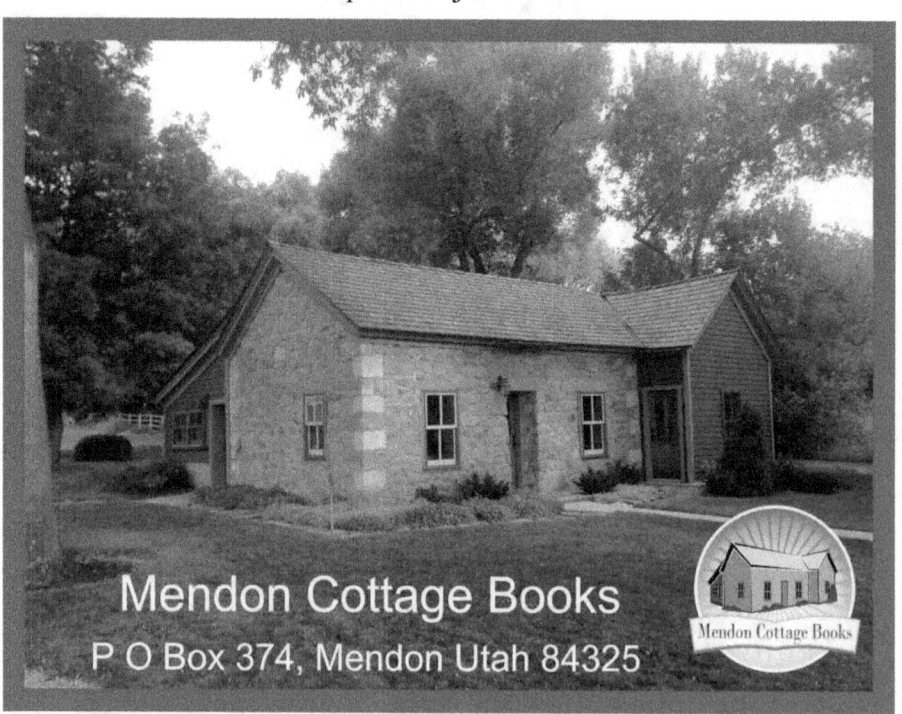

Mendon Cottage Books

P O Box 374, Mendon Utah 84325